Thriver, Not Si
How to Beat Chronic
Fatigue Syndrome

MIGUEL BAUTISTA

ISBN: 9798824067200

DEDICATION

This book is dedicated to all the people who suffer from Chronic Fatigue Syndrome, Myalgic Encephalomyelitis., and Hypersensitive Nervous System Disorders. I was once in your shoes, so I understand how difficult it is to live with a "mystery illness." I hope the content in this book provides inspiration, clarity, and actionable steps that will help change your life for the better like they did for me. I wish you nothing but the best on this journey of health. After recovering and going through this myself, I feel it is my ethical obligation to get this information to as many people as possible.

TABLE OF CONTENTS

ACKNOWLEDGMENTS

I would not be here today if it weren't for the people who supported me throughout this journey. To my family and friends, thank you for encouraging me and staying by my side through all the dark times and helping me rebuild my life into what it is today.

To my handful of friends who constantly checked in on me (you know who you are) to see how I was doing, thank you for helping me keep in touch with the outside world when it felt like everything was slipping away. I appreciate all the times you brought me to doctors' appointments, brought me food to cheer me up, and even just spent time to chat for a couple hours when you could have been in so many other places

To my parents, thank you for always believing in me no matter what and supporting me in my dreams and aspirations. Even if the path was completely different from everyone else, you encouraged me to pursue my dreams with everything I have and to think bigger always, never to settle. You taught me to believe that anything is possible with hard work and determination.

To Lisa, thank you for the unconditional love and support you gave me throughout my recovery journey. I'll never forget counting down the days to seeing you and looking forward to our calls every night when you checked in on me. You were one of the few people I could talk to about everything I was feeling who actually made me feel heard and understood. I have never felt more loved by someone than I did during those dark periods, and many times when I wanted to give up, I would think about how much more life we still needed to experience.

To my grandma and grandpa (rest in peace), thank you for looking after me when I was bedridden for over 6 months and needed 24/7 care. You worked as a team to cook healthy meals every single day, helped me bathe, brush my teeth, spoon-fed me, gave me foot massages whenever I experienced extreme pain and fatigue, and constantly reminded me that everything was going to be ok, no matter how bad my situation seemed.

Thank you to my doctor. Without you I don't believe I would have ever discovered all the tools needed to recover.

I want to thank all of you for believing in me when I did not believe in myself. Sometimes in life we need that extra encouragement, whether from family, friends, or people online to help get us through difficult times. I honestly don't know what would have happened if I didn't have these people in my life at the time.

Introduction

On March 2nd, 2018, I found myself at Richmond General Hospital at twenty two years old. As I rolled my wheelchair into the glass room to meet my doctor for the very first time, I was filled with a mix of excitement, hope, fear, and desperation. I probably looked like a deer in the headlights, because up to this point I had seen at least twenty different doctors, specialists, and alternative doctors in the previous few years. Even though I had literally dozens of horrible symptoms like chronic pain, migraines, heart palpitations, and shortness of breath, I had been told over and over again that I was "normal." I leaned back in my wheelchair behind a large wooden table in what seemed to be a meeting room for doctors and families. "I wonder what this guy's going to tell me this time," I asked myself. Was this going to be another letdown? Were they just going to force me to stand up and start walking around?

After a few minutes he walked in, we shook hands and introduced ourselves.

Then he looked at me, and I'll never forget the first words he spoke. With a grin on his face, he said, "You're going to be fine, just watch. Three months from now you'll be back out in the world walking around like a normal person. What do you think?"

To say I was stunned is an understatement. Other doctors had called me "normal" before, but this time, it sounded more like a promise than a dismissal. I remember looking at him in both disbelief and relief because this was the first time a medical doctor told me they knew how exactly what was going on and that I was going to be ok.

"No way, really? You think so? Even as bad as I am right now? I haven't walked around in almost a year and you really believe I'll do all that?" I replied. "Oh yes, absolutely. You'll be fine living your life again. What do you think?" he said.

It was at that moment something clicked in my mind and my life trajectory changed forever. It felt like an internal switch was flipped. This big, heavy, unbearable burden of being sick seemed ten times lighter, and for the first time, I actually saw a way out of this mystery illness. I had tried to tell myself thousands of times that I would get better - I meditated, did brain retraining exercises, visualized myself getting better, and wrote affirmations for years, but I never truly believed I could actually get better until that moment. For the next twenty minutes we continued our conversation. I asked him how he knew I would get better, who he had helped before me, what did he think was happening and why I felt like I was plugged into an electrical socket 24/7. Every time he answered I felt more and more confident that this was going to work, and I hung onto every single word he said as if he was giving me the cheat codes to beat this level in a video game I had been stuck on for years. I was so desperate just to live a somewhat normal life that I took every single word he said to heart, I was 100 percent committed and onboard— to be honest, when I look back on those moments, if he asked me to get up and walk across the room I probably would have done it without a thought.

Now, that would not have been the right thing to do at that moment (as you'll learn in the coming chapters), but that's how much I trusted him. For the next three and a half weeks, we would meet almost every day to discuss various concepts like what my recovery would look like, the specifics of what I needed to do, what was actually happening within my body to make me feel this way, and so much more. I would sit back in my wheelchair amazed as he drew these charts on the board, made analogies, and broke down complex ideas into the simplest terms. I would also write these concepts down on blank pieces of paper to make sure I retained all of the information. Every day he would teach me a new concept and I would write everything down, adding in my own analogies and examples until I had dozens of pages worth of notes, all breaking down *exactly* how I was going to fully recover. In essence, he gave me the blueprint to recovery.

Luckily, I was open to receiving that blueprint and absorbing the knowledge like a sponge.

One of the many pages of notes I scribbled to remember everything he was teaching me.

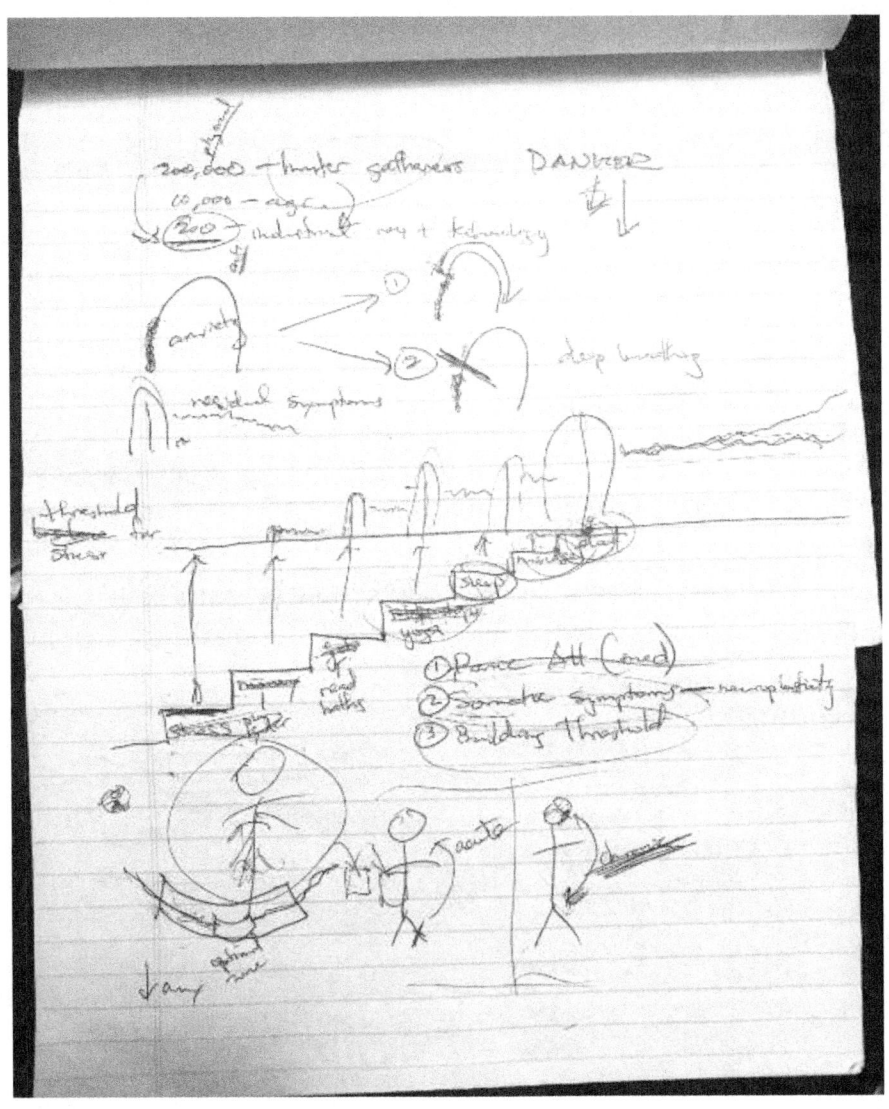

Over the next three and a half years I put these principles into practice, seeing noticeable improvements month after month. Even though symptoms didn't go away overnight, and there were times when I definitely questioned if this was really going to work, I stayed the course and followed the plan, always referring back to my handwritten notes from my stay at the hospital. It was something that I could turn to that helped keep me on track and eventually get to the point where I was not only walking but running a few miles at a time and exercising regularly.

My intention with this book is not only to show you what is possible when it comes to recovering from a hypersensitive nervous system issue but also what the journey looks like on your way to getting your life back. Use this as a tool, refer back to it regularly, and put these concepts into practice. Read (or listen) to this over and over again until the concepts and frameworks are internalized.

If you're reading this right now then you've probably been struggling with CFS (aka a hypersensitive nervous system) for quite some time, and you might feel like there's no hope for recovery. But I'm here to tell you that it is totally possible to overcome this debilitating condition and get your life back. If you're struggling to digest even the thought and possibility of actually recovering and beating this, take it from me. Exactly four short years ago (at the time of writing this) I was in the hospital wondering if I would ever be able to walk again, let alone live a "normal" life. I was being spoon-fed because I had so many symptoms that I felt paralyzed. Sitting up in bed felt equivalent to going up a flight of stairs, just turning over in bed would make the room spin, and often times I felt painful burning sensations whenever I was touched. This was after battling symptoms for years, working on and off, saying no to social events, and putting what felt like my entire life on hold.

The contrast between my current life and where it was then is so vast that I sometimes can't even believe I lived like that for a period of time, but pictures and videos always remind me it wasn't all just a nightmare. It actually happened. But we'll dive more into my story later. For now, I just want you to temporarily suspend your beliefs about what you *think* is going on with your body and absorb the information in this e-book with an open mind. The more open-minded you are when it comes to learning this information, the more you will be able to soak up the knowledge, which can help accelerate your recovery. Also, keep in mind that not everything may apply to your current situation. These are things I found to be true and useful in my recovery that may not be true for you.

Throughout the rest of this book, I'm going to share some tips, strategies, and resources that have helped me recover on my journey as well as some mistakes that can keep people stuck for years (and in some cases decades).

Who this book is for

I want to make it clear that it is absolutely essential for you to do the proper testing to rule out any other potential health issues. When it comes to an illness like this, you're looking for an answer that clearly explains why you're feeling the way you're feeling. I'm not talking about finding out you have bad digestive issues or that you're allergic to certain foods because that doesn't fully explain this level of discomfort.

This book was written for people who experience fatigue, strange symptoms, and/or chronic pain at a level that keeps them from participating in normal activities (getting groceries, minor physical activities, social events...etc.). This is for people who have already seen multiple doctors and specialists, have received multiple negative tests, and have been told...

"Just get some rest..."

"Give it some time and you might get better..."

Or have flat out told you, "We don't know what's wrong..."

If you've had multiple tests done and doctors still have not found anything that explains your symptoms, then this information is for you.

If you've just recently discovered that you might have CFS, have been trying to recover for a while but can't seem to make any progress, or if you've already been making slow progress over time, this book can help you take your recovery to the next level.

Who this book is not for

If you have a severe, diagnosed, incurable condition then this is not for you.

This is not a "get better overnight" book. It was NOT designed to help you regenerate energy and get rid of symptoms quickly enough to go to a wedding next week. That kind of "quick fix" solution does not exist and is often an empty promise from people who cannot help you.

The people who have the highest probability of recovery are Thrivers who are ready to do the work and are willing to learn new concepts - they do not toss the ideas aside if they don't "make a night and day difference" right from day one.

Rewiring your nervous system so it functions normally again takes time and effort. These are concepts that require your commitment to put in the work needed to create change in your recovery journey.

How To Read This Book

There are a lot of books about myalgic encephalomyelitis or chronic fatigue syndrome (CFS) out there. This is not one of them.

This book is not about medical theories or scientific explanations for CFS. It's about recovering from CFS.

You cannot cure CFS by attacking each symptom one at a time. You need to treat this as one big problem, a hypersensitive nervous system issue.

This book will show you how to do that. It will teach you how to calm down your hypersensitive nervous system and stay in a more relaxed, calm, less anxious state than the one you're probably in right now.

This book is not only a guide to chronic fatigue syndrome, but it is also a testimony of my own journey. It contains all the main principles I have learned in order to help people on their own recovery journey. The information in this book is based on personal experience and implementation that worked for me and others, making it a reliable source of information for people experiencing these symptoms.

I am not a doctor, and I cannot diagnose or treat chronic fatigue syndrome, but what I can do is show you the simple steps in the recovery process that I myself used to go from being completely bedridden in the hospital to hiking up a mountain in Hawaii just eleven months later. (See the photos below.)

FEBRUARY 2018   **JANUARY 2019**

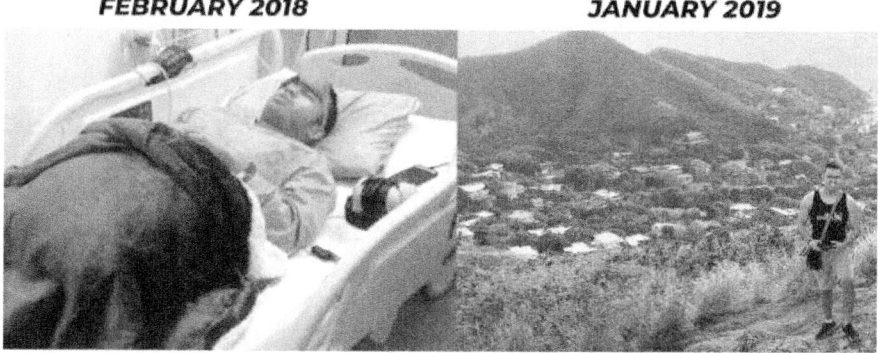

If you've read up to this point, it means you're ready to take the next step in your chronic fatigue syndrome recovery journey. By taking action and reading this e-book, you are already ahead of so many people who suffer from chronic fatigue syndrome and don't even know it is possible to recover. What I ask of you is to not just skim through the information in this book. Read over it, memorize it, and internalize it to the best of your ability.

Pro Tip:

If you want to learn faster and retain more information, try listening to the audiobook while reading the physical book or e-book. This will help store the contents in more places in your brain and improve your understanding of the information. (I've found this to be very helpful.) If you want to pick up an audiobook version, it's available on Amazon or audible.com! If you find the information in this chapter valuable, you may also want to try this "hack" that I used to help me stay focused. Listening to the audiobook while reading helped me keep my attention focused on the material. Try it yourself and see if it works for you!

How Most People Get Sick

I was just a regular kid who loved playing outside. I grew up in Vancouver BC, I had one brother, and I was always a class clown. I loved being active and playing sports, I felt like I just couldn't sit still. I was very driven, almost too driven growing up for my own good. I remember sitting in class one day. I had just gotten my first ever C+ in social studies, and I felt like I had let myself down. I always got straight A's, so how did I let this one grade slip up? I was better than that. C+? That might as well have been a big F on my page. I vowed to myself never again to feel that disappointment in the future, so I became this person who did whatever it took to "succeed." Fast forward several years, and this internal drive led to a very fruitful career early in my life. At twenty-two years old I was one of the top-selling personal trainers in a company with over three hundred trainers, I was driving a nice car, and I was making decent money. On the outside, it might have looked like I had an awesome life, but my body just could not keep up with the demand I was placing on it, and when it came to health I fell into a hole that was so deep I never thought I'd escape. At first, I felt run down, so I forced myself to refocus and stay on track to hit all my goals. Every single morning and night I would rewrite my goals and add onto my never-ending to-do list. After all, I was on a mission for this so-called "success." As the months went on, symptoms became more and more intense until it got so bad I had to go on sick-leave several times.

Like you, I went to dozens and dozens of doctors, specialists, and various medical professionals only to be passed around like a hot potato for years. I was told I could potentially have this illness, that illness, "maybe it's adrenal fatigue," and "maybe it's your thyroid," so over the course of four and a half years I did various treatments.

Some of the receipts from all my treatments with my local naturopath.

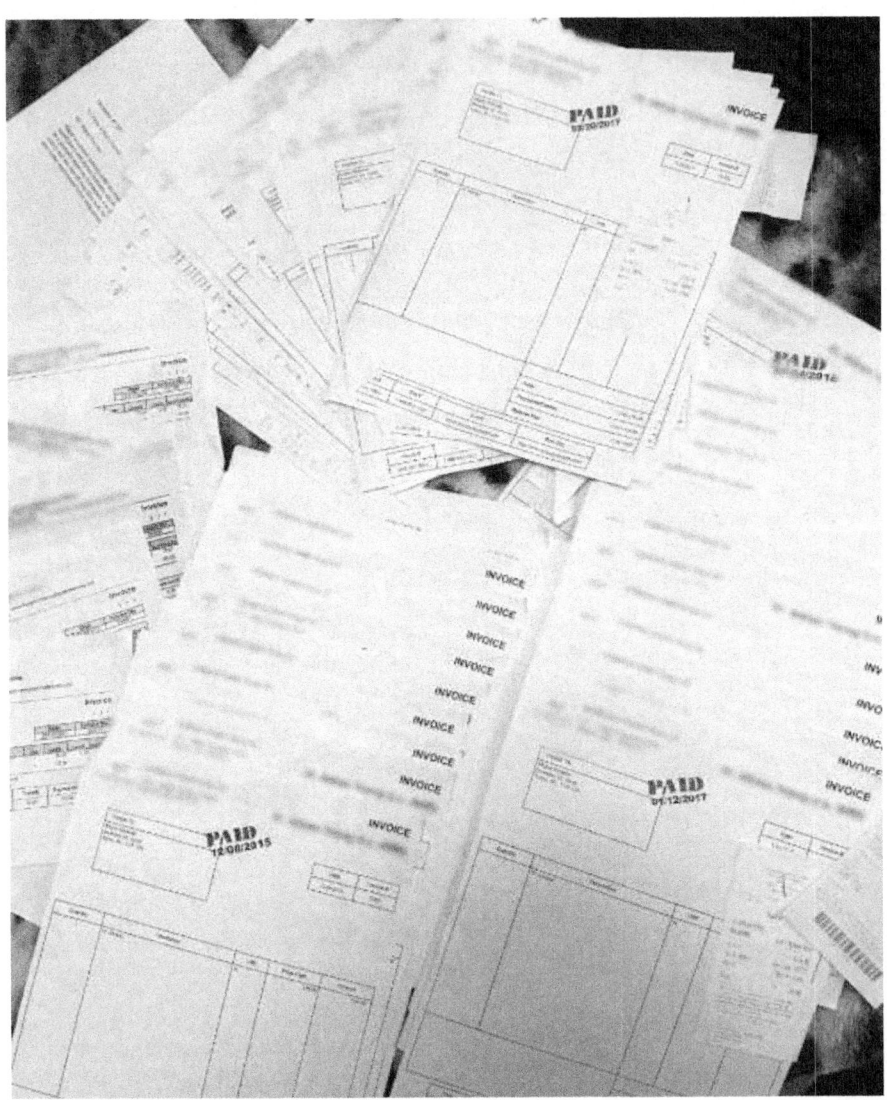

These included multiple detoxes, close to one hundred IV drip treatments, naturopathic supplements, hydrocortisone, thyroid medication, acupuncture for my energy, chiropractic appointments for my headaches, and the list goes on and on.

You might be in the same boat I was in, and maybe you've tried or are currently trying different treatments to beat this mystery illness. For me, even though many of those treatments would help in the short term, none of the benefits had a lasting effect, and over the years my health continued to decline. I had tried adrenal supplements, diets, detoxes, energy supplements, acupuncture, chiropractor, massage therapy, naturopathic medicine, physical therapy, IV therapy, and every time there was a new treatment, I would cross my fingers, hope, and pray that this would be the magic fix that gets me out of this mess. I remember, each Christmas I'd be sitting with family as everyone was opening presents and thinking to myself, "Well, next year I'll be back, stronger than ever, and I'll be able to enjoy the holidays without headaches, food sensitivities, and a host of other symptoms." But the next year would come, and I would still have those headaches, fatigue, and various symptoms that wouldn't allow me to truly enjoy these precious moments.

Frustration was an understatement because it's not like I was rolling over and giving up. If you're reading this, then you can probably relate to what I'm saying.

At twenty-three years old, I was lying in that hospital bed all alone unable to even sit up. People in the bed next to me were being told they had 4 months to live, getting out of surgery, and I just thought to myself, "How did I end up here in such a dark place…?" I thought to myself, "I'm in so deep of a hole, I don't know if I'm ever going to be able to get out." I felt like I had sunk too deep into the quicksand that it was impossible to escape.

Like you, I felt trapped. And like you, I told myself things like:

- No matter what I do, I'm not getting better.
- Every time I try to do activities, I feel so many symptoms.
- I've tried everything. I don't think I'm ever going to get better.
- I'm just stuck at home and missing out on life.
- I feel like I'm going crazy.

Everyone is telling you that you're crazy. I'm telling you that you're not. I'm telling you that what you're going through is real and it's not all in your head. Essentially, when you reach your stress limit, *the body begins to rebel by stopping you from going out into the world.* I'll break that down in the coming chapters.

First, we must become crystal clear on what CFS is.

What is Chronic Fatigue Syndrome?

It's important to note that **for the most part**, in the medical community, the cause and treatment of CFS are unknown. If you were to google chronic fatigue syndrome right now (and I'm sure you've done this many times in the past), it's extremely hard to find an actual solution to the problem, and if you do want to find one, you would have to dig deep and hope to come across channels like mine that offer solutions. Most of the information online just spreads these ideas about how people with CFS are forever doomed or how they'll have to live with this for the rest of their lives.

In this book, we're going to view chronic fatigue syndrome from a different perspective. We're going to use the terms "CFS" and "hypersensitive nervous system issue" interchangeably because it is highly likely that this is what we're dealing with (as long as your tests and scans from doctors for other conditions have come back negative).

Did you know that chronic fatigue syndrome is considered a neurological disorder? This means that the core problem is classified as an issue with the nervous system and not with muscles or joints like so many people think.

The nervous system is responsible for controlling all of the activities in your body, from making your heart beat to digesting your food. When people are experiencing these mystery symptoms seemingly at random, all it means is their nervous system is not functioning optimally.

One of the main reasons why chronic fatigue syndrome is so hard to recover from is because people tend to approach it as if they have multiple problems. They try to fix each individual symptom instead of looking at the problem as a whole.

In many cases, people who identify as having chronic fatigue syndrome (also known as myalgic encephalomyelitis or ME) actually just have a hypersensitive nervous system. This means that the fight-or-flight response is always activated, even when there is no threat.

Some common misconceptions about CFS:

1) A skeptical person might say that *people with chronic fatigue syndrome are just lazy* or that they are making up their symptoms. When people look at you, you'll look perfectly fine physically, but what you feel inside tells a completely different story.

People with chronic fatigue syndrome are not lazy, and they are not making up their symptoms. Many people suffer from chronic fatigue syndrome, and it is a real and serious condition. A hypersensitive nervous system can cause a lot of problems that are masked as many other health problems.

2) If you are like most people with chronic fatigue syndrome, you have probably been told by your doctor that *there is nothing wrong with you.* You may feel like you are fighting a battle against your own body. Doctors often do not know how to diagnose or treat chronic fatigue syndrome, leaving patients feeling lost and alone. Some skeptics may say that chronic fatigue syndrome cannot be healed. They might say that it is a lifelong condition with no known cure. This book will show you that this is not the case.

3) *Recovery is impossible.* You don't have to let chronic fatigue syndrome rule the rest of your life - you can take back control and start improving today. In fact, you'll hear from many people who have fully recovered that on the other side of this journey they have a newfound appreciation and gratitude towards life. Through all the trials and tribulations during the illness, we are tested physically, mentally, emotionally, and most of all, spiritually. We are pushed to the very edge of our limits, which only makes us stronger. It's kind of like how a beautiful samurai sword is created - it's placed in extreme heat, taken out of the fire, hammered, folded, cooled, and this cycle is repeated thousands of times. At the end of it all is a beautiful, one-of-a-kind piece of art. You may not see it now, but when you're better, on the other side of this dark journey, you'll see that all this suffering had a purpose, and along the journey, there were valuable lessons that you would have never learned if all this didn't happen.

Breaking Down The Science

How Our (Sympathetic) Nervous System Functions

We need to understand what's happening in the body because we can't fix something if we don't know *what* to fix. The main concept I want to talk about here is the stress threshold, but before we even get into that, we're going to talk about how the brain was designed to function from a *survival standpoint*.

- For 200,000 years, humans were hunter-gatherers - primed for exposing themselves to physical danger in order to survive. We were *wired and designed* to look for danger around us. (There was a high level of physical danger back then).

- For 10,000-20,000 years there was the agricultural revolution - we no longer had to expose ourselves to high levels of real danger in order to survive. There was a LARGE decrease in danger.

- For the last 100 years, there has been a technology revolution - real danger has been DRASTICALLY decreased.

Have a look at this timeline to see how recent these massive technological changes in our lives have been.

HUMAN TIMELINE

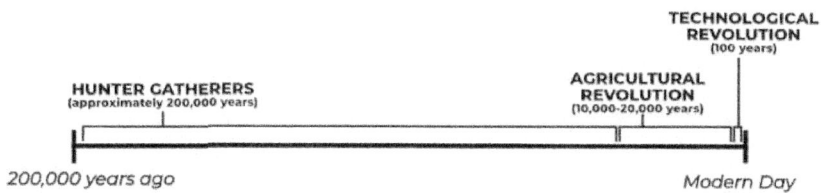

As you can see, for tens of thousands of years our brains have been primed to look for stressors in our life. Today, our brains often think we are in physical danger and that there are threats around, even though that may not be the case. This is important in understanding why you feel pain and other symptoms.

The stress response is a bodily reaction that occurs when the brain perceives a threat. The body releases hormones such as adrenaline and cortisol to help us deal with the threat. This is called the fight-or-flight response.

The fight-or-flight response was originally designed to help us survive in dangerous situations, but nowadays it's often triggered by things that are not life-threatening, such as stress at work, traffic jams, arguments, public speaking, financial problems - the list goes on and on.

If the fight-or-flight response is activated too often, it can lead to a chronic increase in cortisol levels. Cortisol is a hormone that's released when the body is under stress. It plays an important role in helping the body deal with stressful situations, but if it's elevated for long periods, it can have harmful effects on the body. For example, it can cause the heart to beat faster, brain fog, palpitations, anxiety, panic attacks, dizziness, vertigo, fatigue, blood sugar issues, and more.

When we are constantly stressed, our health suffers.

The Stress Threshold

Our bodies have a baseline for stress - *a stress threshold*. Stress can be mental, emotional, financial, and it can be related to family, work, diet, relationships, etc. As stressors (and *perceived stressors*) are added to life, our stress threshold becomes smaller and smaller. Once stressors push your nervous system over the threshold, you begin to experience symptoms. This implies that persistent stress can cause pain and symptoms even if the original stressor has been resolved. This is because the nervous system has become sensitized to stress and now reacts to seemingly minor stressors as if they were major threats.

Your primal brain's main job is to keep you alive. When stressors become too intense, they can be seen as a danger to the brain. (Work stress can be perceived as seeing a snake, a car beeping its horn can be perceived as a war cry, losing a video game can make us feel like we just lost a valuable opportunity).

When we are constantly overexerting ourselves physically and mentally, we are always going to be operating above our stress threshold. That's when we start to feel symptoms. We are going way too hard, way too fast, and adding too much stress overall. When we stack stress on our nervous system, it can get to the point where our brain places limiters on our body - those limiters are fatigue and pain. *From a psychological perspective, the high amount of stress and symptoms WILL lead to heightened anxiety and fear.*

Most of the time what happens is we become trapped in this *vicious cycle of symptoms* leading to more anxiety + more anxiety leading to more symptoms. This can keep us stuck for years because things just spiral downwards and little to no progress is made. It might feel impossible to reverse this cycle of symptoms and anxiety.

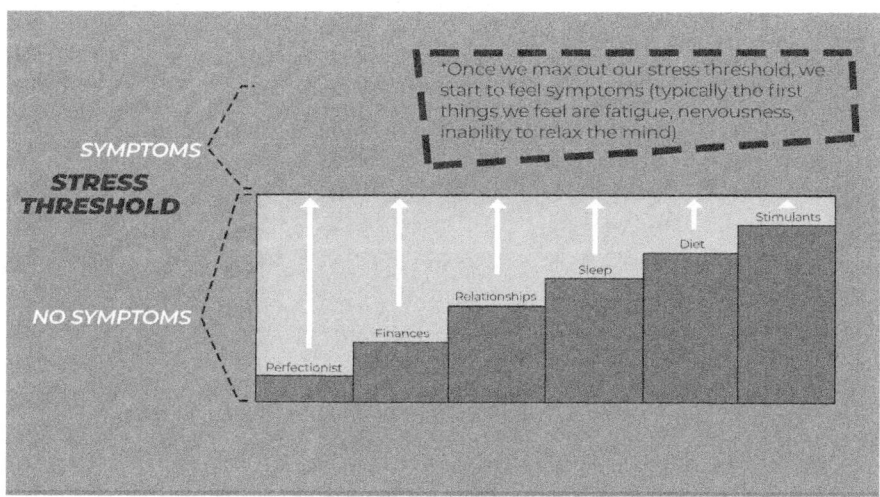

The good news is that there are ways to break out of this downward spiral. By learning about the hypersensitive nervous system and how it contributes to CFS, we can start to make changes in our lives that will help us recover. There is hope for a better future – we just need to take the first step. We'll learn more about breaking out of the downward spiral next.

ASK YOURSELF

What are some stressors in your life that have caused you to go over the stress threshold? The more aware you are about what caused all this, the more likely you will avoid falling into those same habits.

Identify at least 15 physical or mental habits that led you on this path. If you're not fully aware of how you got here, you will stay stuck and continue to make the same mistakes.

Ex.

<u>Mental Thought Habits:</u>

- If I do more things, then I will get better.
- I fixate on unrealized potential outcomes.
- I always have to be doing something or keep busy.
- My mind puts a spotlight on problems (including other people's problems.)
- Am I ever actually going to fully recover?

<u>Physical Habits:</u>

- Not getting enough sleep
- Eating junk food
- Taking too many stimulants (coffee, energy drinks, supplements, etc.)
- Trying to do more activities every time I have a little bit of energy

The Downward Spiral - Why and How People STAY Stuck

Typically, *what causes* people to become sick with CFS is *not what keeps them sick*. This is why people can stay sick for years because even though the major stressors are long gone, the symptoms stick around and often get even worse. We must become aware of the downward spiral that's easy to get stuck in. It looks like this:

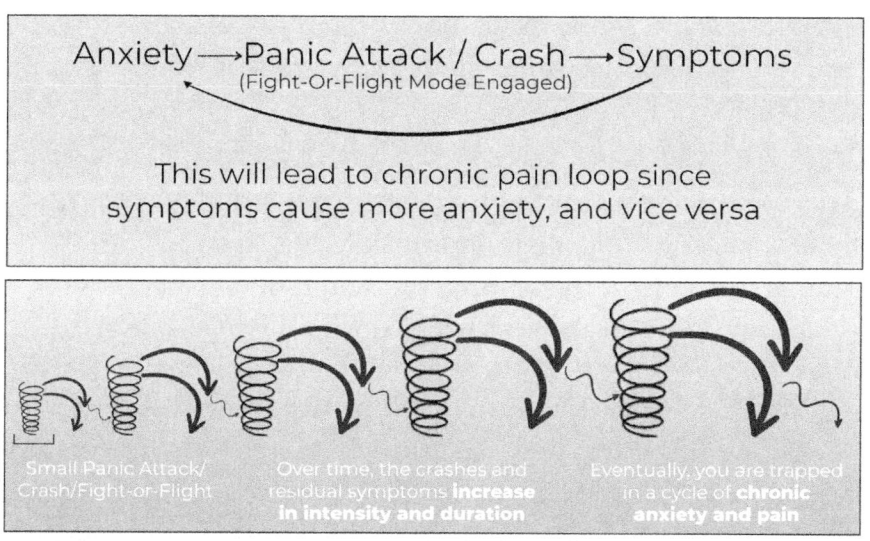

The main issue with most people is that they get trapped in a downward spiral.

This keeps them stuck feeling like they're running in circles making no progress. The goal is to focus on the hypersensitive nervous system, the root cause, and work from there.

When people are first diagnosed or come to the conclusion via process of elimination that they have chronic fatigue syndrome (CFS), they often feel lost and overwhelmed. This is understandable, as CFS can manifest itself in several different ways, and it can be difficult to find a treatment that works. Many people try numerous different treatments and supplements before finding one that helps. However, this approach can be counterproductive, as it keeps the person stuck in a cycle of trial and error. This kind of desperation made me jump from treatment to treatment, spending thousands of dollars and doing anything I could to gain traction. Before I knew it, I had multiple different doctors telling me five different things, giving me five different tools from five different practices. Then, it got to the point where I gave up on doctors and the medical system because nobody was giving me solid answers or solutions to my problems.

I remember working with a naturopath because at the time he was the only medical professional who seemed to be putting in an effort to explore what could be causing all my symptoms. For two years we treated what I had as adrenal fatigue, so I was taking adaptogens, adrenal supplements, and doing Myer's cocktail IV treatments regularly. Every week I'd show up to the office, swipe my credit card, and cross my fingers that whatever we were doing was working. Sure, some weeks felt better than others and the treatments helped temporarily, but every twelve months I just seemed to be getting worse, and every Christmas, every birthday, every summer I was able to do less and less until it got to the point where I was completely bedridden. As many people with CFS experience, when treatments didn't work, I just became more hopeless and desperate for solutions.

It can be overwhelming trying to figure out where to start, however, it's important to remember that CFS is essentially a hypersensitive nervous system issue. This means that the main goal of treatment should be to calm the nervous system down, not fix individual symptoms (as long as there are no other underlying health issues). Once the nervous system starts to shift out of a state of fight-or-flight, the symptoms of CFS will begin to lift. The most important thing is to stay focused on the underlying causes and not get stuck in a downward spiral of anxiety and panic about symptoms. The goal is to focus on *ONE problem*, the hypersensitive nervous system, and work from there.

Now that we understand how we got here and what keeps most people stuck - we have to figure out how to get out.

I had an epiphany that looking back, knowing what I know now, recovery from CFS can be broken down into a very simple process. There are dozens and dozens of treatments, coping mechanisms, and tactics out there. Some work and some don't, and most of them are exactly that - coping mechanisms (aka short-term solutions that don't actually fix the problem). Regardless of how you move forward in your recovery, this is what I know to be true. There are THREE things that need to happen for a full recovery.

1. THE MINDSHIFT

2. PROPERLY DEALING WITH SYMPTOMS

3. BUILDING THRESHOLD

THE MINDSHIFT

Back when I was sick, what I didn't realize was that everyone who I was going to for help was looking at this whole problem from one perspective. They were chasing down every single symptom I was feeling. Of course, heart palpitations and postural tachycardia syndrome (POTS) symptoms led me to cardiologists, while chronic pain and tingling led me to neurologists. The health anxiety and loss of identity led me to psychologists, and the low energy led me to endocrinologists thinking it was adrenal fatigue-related. I was doing everything I could, researching and booking appointments with specialists in different cities, driving hundreds of kilometres just to hear "you're normal," or "just get some rest." Eventually, as I continued to decline, things got so bad that I had to live with my grandparents for six months, where they helped feed and bathe me because I was in such bad shape I couldn't do it myself. Then, as if that wasn't bad enough, my symptoms were so severe that I found myself in the intensive care unit at my local hospital thinking there was no way of coming back from this. I had officially hit rock bottom...or so I thought.

I still remember that first night being transferred to the hospital. I was so scared because I thought my body would just shut down from all the stimuli. The sound of the ambulance, the bright hospital lights, people being rushed in and out of rooms beside me... It was very different from what I was used to experiencing in my quiet room during the previous six months.

For weeks, I woke up to the sounds of machines beeping and having my blood pressure taken. "Good morning, what's your name? When's your birthday? Any pain or discomfort?" they'd ask me every day precisely at eight am. I still remember exactly how my IV machines would beep whenever an air bubble got stuck, as well as the smell of the cleaning agents they ran through the air filters. They had done various scans, blood tests, and assessments and brought many specialists in to try and figure out what was going on with me with no success. After about three and a half weeks of hell (which felt like three months), they finally told me that based on the scans everything checked out normal and I was approved to be discharged.

However, there was this one doctor they wanted to introduce me to who could *potentially* fix me. Since I was in somewhat stable condition at this point, but still not able to sit up or get out of the hospital without experiencing excruciating pain and waves of intense symptoms, they told me I had two options.

Option one: they could call my dad, who would pick me up, and I would be sent home, where I would be an outpatient. This meant that I'd have to come back to the hospital regularly to meet with this new doctor. Immediately I knew I couldn't go with option one because I couldn't even get into a wheelchair, the thought of being transported back and forth to the hospital regularly was not even a doable option in my mind, so option one was off the list.

Option two, however, would allow me to stay at the hospital and work with my doctor daily. There was one catch though: *the only extra rooms that were available were in the psychiatric ward.* "They can't be serious," I thought to myself. A psych ward? I wasn't crazy, I wasn't making this up, and what were they going to do anyways that could possibly help? Force me to stand up, walk around, and tell me it's all in my head? I've seen how it goes in the movies and didn't want that label of being crazy or out of my mind.

I had a few minutes to make a decision, but I knew I really only had one option. "If I don't like it there, can I go home at any time?" I asked. "Oh yes, you would stay there voluntarily, so you could go home at any time," the nurse replied. I took a deep breath and finally gave in. "I'll do it," I told the nurse.

I was terrified, nervous, excited, and curious about what to expect. A part of me was fighting the urge to tell them to just send me home, but I knew I couldn't go back to a life of just surviving. My desire to get better outweighed the fear of being placed in that *particular* section of the hospital, and I had to fix this once and for all.

What happened over the next month was nothing short of a miracle.

A New Opportunity

It wasn't until they paired me up with a doctor who truly understood what was going on that my life turned around. Despite all of my attempts to get better over the years and failing, luckily I was paired up with a new doctor who said that the solution to all of this was focusing on **fixing one main problem - rewiring my nervous system out of a hypersensitive state.**

When people are first diagnosed with chronic fatigue syndrome (CFS), or even if they've come to that conclusion by process of elimination through various tests, they often feel like they have been struck by some freak, incurable illness. They may feel like they have multiple problems, and that each problem requires its own solution. However, this is not the case. Instead of focusing on fixing each symptom, one needs to focus on getting the nervous system back into balance between sympathetic and parasympathetic. For example, if someone has pain, you can't just give them pain medication and call it a day. You have to address the root cause of the pain. In almost all instances, once the nervous system is functioning properly again, all of the other symptoms go away on their own.

This means that the main goal of treatment should be to calm the nervous system down. Once the nervous system is no longer in a state of fight-or-flight, the symptoms of CFS will begin to dissipate.

I want to share with you some of the invaluable lessons I've learned on my recovery journey.

Internalizing the Science

When you understand how chronic fatigue syndrome works, it gives you the power to take control of your health. You can start to see the patterns in your symptoms and learn how to better manage them. This is not an easy journey. In fact, it will probably be one of the hardest things you ever go through, but it is so worth it.

There are many helpful resources out there that can teach you about chronic fatigue syndrome, but I encourage you to regularly watch the videos on my YouTube channel as everything I say in the videos feeds into what I share in this book. All the information I share does not conflict from one point to the next. This makes it much easier for you to digest the information since you'll be learning from a consistent source of information rather than multiple sources offering different solutions that contradict each other. I've tried consuming as much information as I could online about the subject of how to recover from CFS, and it only left me more confused the more I watched because each resource would provide me with different solutions. I want you to avoid going down those endless rabbit holes, and I know you know what I'm talking about. The googling, the clicking on random forums and links, then consuming content that totally contradicts what you've read just minutes prior. I'm willing to bet that you've even accidentally come across articles of people saying you can never heal from something like this and then felt hopeless for the next few hours to few days. It's ok, I've made that mistake many times as well. That's why I feel it is my moral obligation to share this information with people like you through all my content online, because I wish someone told me these things when my back was against the wall.

It's important to note that when you truly understand this illness, it changes everything. I mean EVERYTHING. When my doctor shared all this information with me, all the heaviness of fear, panic, and worry lifted because all of a sudden I was confident that I was going to recover. It all clicked, it made sense, and everything he was teaching me answered the basic questions I had asked myself thousands of times prior to meeting him. It was no longer a guessing game, and it really came down to executing the strategies, and when I internalized all these concepts, this new knowledge became a formula that made recovery inevitable. You will no longer feel like you are a victim - instead, you will be in control of your own destiny. You will feel like a Thriver - not a survivor.

Belief - The Thriver Mindset

You need to start thinking of yourself as a Thriver, not just a survivor. When you view yourself in this new light, you will be more motivated to take action and make progress. On YouTube, there are chronic fatigue syndrome communities full of inspiring stories of people who have made incredible recoveries - chronic fatigue syndrome doesn't have to be a life sentence. At the same time, there are even more stories of people saying you can't recover, and this illness will never go away. Which story do you want to believe and pay attention to? Are you a Thriver or a survivor?

In order to recover, you need to let go of any past beliefs that may be holding you back. You may feel like you have tried everything, and nothing has worked. But it is important to keep fighting for your health. Remember, your body is designed to heal itself. It's more resilient than you could ever imagine. You just need to give it the right environment. Trust in the process, and have faith that recovery is possible. There are so many people who have gone through what you are going through and have come out the other side. I've seen the approach I share in this book work for people who have been dealing with this for one year and people who have had this for ten years. I understand that chronic fatigue syndrome can feel incredibly overwhelming and confusing, but don't give up. You are not alone in this journey. There are many people who are rooting for you and want to see you succeed. I am one of them.

Once you *believe* that recovery is possible, things get a lot easier. The path of recovery becomes much clearer and there is less guesswork throughout the entire process. You become more hopeful, positive, and consistent in your efforts because you understand the science behind what's going on. Your old way of thinking might have been something like this: "I don't know what's wrong with me. I feel so exhausted all the time and in so much pain. Nothing seems to help. I feel hopeless, like I'm never going to get better."

Now, with this new belief, your new way of thinking is: "I know exactly what's wrong with me and what I need to do to get better. I just need to stick to the plan."

Setting Realistic Expectations

You have to understand that change is not going to happen overnight. When you understand this, you stay composed in the face of adjustment periods. This is not an easy journey and there are no guarantees, but with time and patience, you can make incredible progress. Healing takes time, and it's important to be patient with yourself during the process. Rome wasn't built in a day, and your health won't be rebuilt overnight either.

One step at a time. That's all you can do, and trust that each step you take is moving you closer to your goal of Thriving health.

The Thriver mindset is about more than just recovering from chronic fatigue syndrome. It's about becoming a whole and healthy person once again. This means that you don't just focus on your physical health, but also your emotional, spiritual, and mental health. You need to address all aspects of yourself in order to move closer to your potential. All of these areas are interconnected and need to be in balance in order for you to feel your best. Wholeness means that you accept yourself – the good and the bad. You don't need to be perfect, you just need to be authentic and real. When you are living your life from a place of wholeness and authenticity, you are more empowered and capable of making a difference in the world.

When you try to focus on too many things at once, it creates a lot of noise and chaos, which can keep you stuck running in circles making no progress. The goal is to focus on ONE problem, the hypersensitive nervous system, and work from there.

How your mindset can stimulate your nervous system

Imagine there's a spider on your table. It's a small spider, it seems harmless, right? Not too scary. You could probably pick it up with a piece of paper towel and bring it outside – or you could take a really powerful magnifying glass and put it over that spider. With that magnifying glass, all of a sudden that spider seems ten times bigger, which means it appears ten times more dangerous, which means you're not getting anywhere near it, and anxiety goes through the roof. *The object did not change, but the lens through which we perceive it did.*

Similarly, when we see symptoms with the thought of "What could this be...what's happening to me???" the symptoms will feel significantly worse due to our nervous system being stimulated with fear and worry.

Having made hundreds of hours worth of videos and talked to hundreds of people since sharing my work online, I know this is the mistake almost everyone makes. They get caught up in negative self-talk and anticipation of triggering symptoms.

You don't want symptoms to rule your life because before you know it, you're going to get stuck in that cycle where all you're thinking about is avoiding them at all costs. Eventually, it gets to the point where you have that 24/7 feeling and live life as if you are walking on eggshells. I was the exact same way. I had to think hard about anything and everything I did to make sure I was hypervigilant about every action. From standing up slowly, to making sure I only walked to the washroom a certain number of times per day to conserve my energy, even to the number of times I rolled over in bed, I became trapped in that mindset of "be extremely careful or you might trigger horrible symptoms."

Most people don't realize that just because we may be physically resting, it does not mean our nervous system is at rest. Our emotions (especially negative emotions like fear and worry) can keep our nervous systems in a state of fight-or-flight.

DEALING WITH SYMPTOMS

The ONE thing that needs to happen in order to create massive positive change

"Your success is determined by how well you respond to symptoms."

My doctor mentioned this to me during every one of our meetings in the hospital. This quote is now burned into my memory, and I truly see it as the core phrase I had to carry with me during my recovery journey.

We need to shift our mindset to see symptoms from a different perspective. We need to see it as an OPPORTUNITY and NOT AS A SETBACK/ CRASH. Having symptoms is ON the way to recovery, not IN the way of recovery.

Having symptoms is a way your nervous system tells you it's overstimulated. We just need to gain trust with our brain and body once again and understand that if we have seen doctors, specialists, run multiple tests and scans, and nothing is showing up to explain how we are feeling, it's more than likely that your body is not in any real danger and is simply overstimulated. Understanding this takes a lot of mystery out of the symptoms and you're able to respond to them with more logic than emotion.

They are not signs that you are doing something wrong or that you are not on the right track - they are simply scientific, primal responses your body is experiencing in response to a stimulus.

Think of symptoms as something that comes and goes - it's temporary. You might have more symptoms sometimes or fewer symptoms other times - it just depends on how much stimulation your nervous system is experiencing.

What most people don't realize is when we fixate on symptoms, our brains start to put a magnifying glass over those symptoms, so they will feel a lot worse. This is why there have probably been times when you did things you did not think you were capable of and were ok, yet there were other times when you did much less yet felt a lot worse. I can almost guarantee you had a high level of anxiety, worry, and fear before, during, and after the situation that was worse.

The deeper you are into this illness and the more discomfort you feel on a daily basis, naturally, you will be in a much more negative mindset. I'm not saying you have to think positive all the time and just ignore what you're feeling in your body. What I am saying is you need to be aware and catch yourself going into that fearful, worrying mindset. As I mentioned earlier, the more you understand what's happening, the less emotional you will be about the symptoms. Also, just because you have little to no fear of symptoms does not mean they're going to just disappear overnight.

It took me several months to completely get over my fear of symptoms, and it was honestly one of the hardest things I've ever had to do in my life. It wasn't easy by any means, but it was so worth it once I finally got to a point where I realized that *I had the power to make my symptoms improve.*

In fact, when I made the shift and stopped fearing them and instead started to see them as opportunities for growth, that's when I saw leaps and bounds in my recovery. I rewired the way I perceived the symptoms. I was no longer living in fear and anticipation of symptoms, but instead focusing on the present moments and what I was able to do that day. My nervous system was no longer constantly stuck in fight-or-flight mode, which meant that I was no longer always on high alert and triggered by the slightest stimulus.

Once we understand this, we can start to see symptoms in a different light. Instead of seeing them as a setback or a crash, we can start to see them as an opportunity -an opportunity to take a break, to rest, rewire, and heal.

Committing to Recovery

Once you shift your mindset and make the conscious decision that you no longer want to stay in this cycle, and you're willing to break free from all the old, hindering thinking patterns, you must practice brain retraining every chance you get. This means that when you feel symptoms, a majority of the time you **should** be redirecting your thoughts to something more positive. Redirect your thoughts to anything but the negative emotions you have about the symptoms (fear, worry, anxiety, panic, depression, etc.). You MUST see episodes of chronic pain as **opportunities** to rewire the brain.

When I got out of the hospital, I would spend a lot of time just sitting outside. I was sitting on a bench overlooking the water and I was feeling some symptoms just from walking 100 metres from the apartment. I no longer felt anger, fear, or frustration towards these symptoms. Instead, I thought to myself, "This is another opportunity to rewire my brain." I welcomed the symptoms and sought them out knowing that the only way to make them go away for good was by redirecting

away from them when they were present. There's this one lady who messaged me online. We spent a few months going back and forth, and I was giving her advice. She was listening, and

every time she would feel that doubt creeping in, she'd shoot me a message. I would remind her that symptoms are expected during recovery, but keep on doing that brain retraining. Just that reassurance made all the difference, and sure enough, about 6 months later she was living her life again. This is the same with people in Recovery Jumpstart, my ONLINE interactive program designed to help people struggling with CFS, Panic Disorder, or a Hypersensitive Nervous System learn how to once and for all overcome the fatigue, pain, and symptoms that come along with the illness.

Sometimes all we need is a little bit of reassurance from someone who understands what we're going through, even if it's a simple "You're going to be ok, you're in an adjustment period."

Adjustment Periods vs. Crashes

Many people confuse a crash with an adjustment period. Most people with CFS will feel some symptoms during this time, such as being very tired for a few days, experiencing headaches, body aches and pains, irritable bowel syndrome (IBS), and a handful of other symptoms. Immediately after this, they may think, "Darn, I'm crashing. I'm going backward, I shouldn't have done this and that...," and they go into this crisis mode. All of a sudden they feel like they've gone back to square one. This isn't usually the case (unless you've really overstimulated your body).

In order to have somewhat of an idea of gauging where you are between the two, I would assume you have an idea of what it's like to "crash," so use the worst crash you've had as a reference to compare the quantity, intensity, and duration of symptoms to.

Have a look at this chart below.

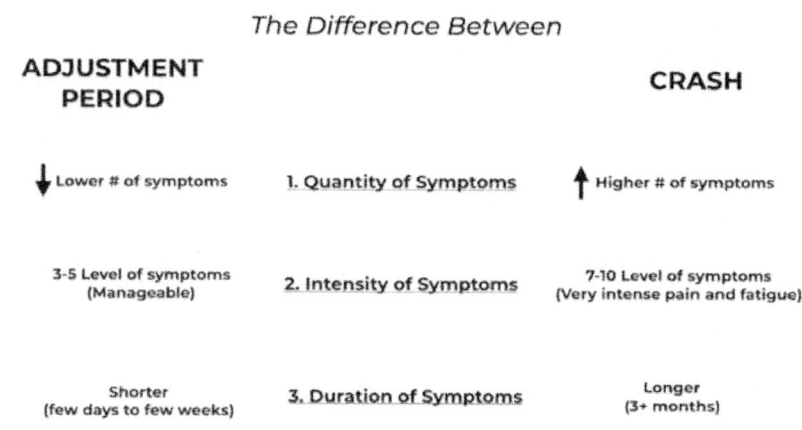

The Difference Between

ADJUSTMENT PERIOD		**CRASH**
↓ Lower # of symptoms	**1. Quantity of Symptoms**	↑ Higher # of symptoms
3-5 Level of symptoms (Manageable)	**2. Intensity of Symptoms**	7-10 Level of symptoms (Very intense pain and fatigue)
Shorter (few days to few weeks)	**3. Duration of Symptoms**	Longer (3+ months)

There are some differences between a crash and an adjustment period, and based on my experience, having gone through hundreds of adjustment periods and dozens of bad "crashes," I've narrowed it down to three areas.

- Quantity of symptoms
- Intensity of symptoms
- Duration of symptoms

Quantity of Symptoms

The quantity of symptoms in an adjustment period is going to be much lower than when in a "crash." Instead of having twenty to thirty potential symptoms, there's only a handful and you feel that these are manageable.

Intensity of Symptoms

The biggest telltale sign to differentiate between which state you are in is the intensity of symptoms. Going back to what I mentioned earlier about using your worst "crash" as a reference, think back to the intensity of symptoms at that time - that will be a ten on our imaginary scale.

If you are in a crash, you are at about seven or higher out of ten. The symptoms are very intense. When symptoms are under a seven, it's pretty safe to consider this an adjustment period.

Duration of Symptoms

During an adjustment, the flare-up of symptoms may last 2-3 days to 2-3 weeks, however in a crash they last longer.

The biggest overall differentiators are these:

Adjustment periods are manageable. With adjustment periods you can still move around and get through the day, it's just very uncomfortable. Nonetheless, you're not completely stuck suffering.

Crashes are extremely difficult to manage. Typically, you're in bed for days if not weeks unable to perform the simplest of tasks.

If you have lots of intense symptoms stacked on top of each other and it's at the point where you don't even want to move for a few weeks, you're likely in a crash, and you need to pull back on everything you're doing. I think the biggest factor for a lot of people is really the intensity of symptoms because that is what affects us the most. Keep in mind this will always be subjective. How much pain and fatigue are we feeling? What is the level of overall discomfort? Sometimes you'll have a very high intensity of symptoms, a very high quantity of symptoms, but most of it goes away within a week. While it *felt* like a "crash," it was actually an adjustment period.

There's no black or white way to tell which you are in, but using this framework can give you at least an idea of where you're at.

For the most part, what I teach in Recovery Jumpstart is you want to have really good periods of time where you're not in a crash and you're not in a major adjustment period. During other times you do want to be in an adjustment period. Think of them as the training grounds where you do the work to re-wire the way you perceive symptoms and retrain your mind that the symptoms are a result of an extreme magnification of stress triggers.

Remember that just because you have symptoms does not mean you are going backward in your recovery. By understanding the difference between a crash and an adjustment period, you can better manage your levels of activity AND mindset.

Digestive Issues and Food Sensitivities

As always, make sure you do proper testing with your doctors to rule out any potential gut issues. If they perform multiple tests and don't find anything that explains your digestive, stomach, or gut symptoms, then you can be pretty confident that this is part of the hypersensitive nervous system issue.

Growing up I never really had digestion issues. I could pretty much eat anything at any time, whether the food contained gluten, sugar, caffeine, dairy, stimulants, or other "bad" ingredients. None of those ever bothered me. However, once I started feeling more fatigued and run-down, I found that I wasn't able to tolerate these same foods and ingredients anymore. I found that the more symptoms I had overall, the more sensitive I was to certain foods. Eventually, it got to a point where I couldn't even tolerate eating a single piece of candy, chocolate, or fried food, and if I did try these foods, I would experience intense symptoms shortly after. Sometimes my heart would race, I'd feel lightheaded, and I'd have to go to the washroom multiple times over the next few hours.

I remember working as a personal trainer one morning, and before our shift, the manager decided to buy everybody some hot chocolate. I quickly drank my small cup of hot chocolate and for the next several hours my heart was pounding. All it took for my heart rate to go from one hundred to about one hundred forty was walking over to different areas of the gym and picking up light weights to hand to my clients. I had to go to the washroom several times during sessions with clients as I experienced cramps and stomach pain.

Another time I was having dinner at a sushi restaurant with friends at a place we'd been to about a dozen times before. We ordered the typical dishes we always enjoyed, sushi rolls, fried chicken, and tempura. Afterward, I drove home as I would on any other night, but after going to sleep I woke up in a panic because my heart felt like it was pounding out of my chest. I immediately had to go to the washroom and the room felt like it was spinning. The symptoms and anxiety levels were ten out of ten. My body was in a state of complete panic.

Over the years, as I continued on that downward spiral of health, I developed a sensitivity to a lot of different foods that got worse over the years. I did multiple tests to look for any potential food intolerances causing these issues, however, nothing ever showed up on the tests. In fact, while working with a naturopath, I even tried doing a couple of detoxes, which ended up doing more harm than good. Not only was my energy completely depleted for the next several weeks, but my food intolerances also got much worse.

Here is how I finally realized that food played a smaller role in my recovery than I thought. (Keep in mind, I didn't have any detectable food intolerances. If you have detectable food intolerances, consult with your doctor for medical advice.)

At my worst, I was completely bedridden living with my grandparents for six months. My grandparents were doing everything they could to try and help me recover, so they would prepare fresh, healthy food every single day. I was eating eggs, salads, sweet potatoes, avocados, and high-quality proteins along with other "healthy foods," yet I continued to feel worse (more pain, symptoms, and fatigue). I was stuck in a 24/7 cycle of adjustment periods. Even though I was eating healthy foods and cutting out all junk foods, I was still experiencing upset stomachs, especially during adjustment periods. Eventually, I moved to the hospital and after about a month of tests, treatments, and medications, I met my doctor who helped me understand what was going on and how to make these symptoms go away for good. When I met him, we didn't try to treat my headaches, high heart rate, shortness of breath, food insensitivities, and the other dozen symptoms I was experiencing at the time. We just focused on treating one thing - my hypersensitive nervous system.

To my surprise, I started improving in different areas. Not only were my symptoms less intense, but my gut actually started being able to tolerate different foods. I remember my friend visited me one time in the hospital. He dropped off several snacks and cookies, and at the time I hadn't eaten a cookie in probably one year at that point. I tried eating a cookie...no adjustment period triggered. I had a cookie each day for the next several days without experiencing gut issues.

What really shocked me was the fact that I couldn't even tolerate any of these foods just a month prior. In fact, I could barely tolerate anything. That's actually what put me in the hospital, my inability to digest food, because I would throw it up or have extremely uncomfortable stomach issues.

When I started introducing these foods into my diet again, not only was I NOT getting worse, or even staying the same, I just kept getting better. This is the ultimate example that really proved to me that this was more than an issue with my diet. Having the ability to enjoy good food is one of the things people look forward to when I ask them what they envision their life to be like after they recover.

A lot of people say, "If I could just eat a slice of pizza...if I could just eat my favourite candy...if I could just enjoy a really nice meal and not have to worry about what happens after, I'd be happy." What I tell a lot of people is not only can that be possible, but it will happen sooner than they think. For a majority of people who join <u>Recovery Jumpstart</u>, within two to three months they are able to start enjoying foods they had to avoid for so long because their nervous system is able to tolerate more stimuli.

For me, it was really nice to know that I didn't have to avoid these foods forever, which is what I had started to believe. I thought I'd never be able to enjoy amazing food again or take part in delicious meals at social events without worrying about the food completely wiping me out for the next few days.

When the body is in a state of fight-or-flight, much of our blood supply goes to the "attack" and "defence" muscles. The body is preparing to fight or flee, so all the blood needs to be in our arms and legs in order to help us stay alive when danger is lurking. In this state, the priority is not digestion. This is why when we're more anxious it's more difficult for our bodies to digest food. There's not enough blood flow to the digestive organs to function optimally. The body is focused on fight, flight, or freeze, not so much on resting and digesting. This explains why, especially when you're feeling extra anxious, wired, or like your body is buzzing with anticipation of something, we tend to experience more upset stomach and digestive issues.

Maybe you're in an adjustment period, and you're upset that you can't move around and do all these things that you used to do, and you start getting down on yourself. All this puts you in a state of stress, and we know that stress leads to symptoms. Having those symptoms can upset you even more, which makes you more stressed, which leads to more IBS symptoms, and you can see how this whole thing can snowball and get out of control.

Today I'm very grateful I have the ability to enjoy all the foods I like especially on vacations where food options are unpredictable. I have a special appreciation for food because I was deprived of a lot of it for so long. Although the goal is not to eat unhealthily and go all out on junk food when you get better, the goal is to have the freedom of options and choices for things that you can eat.

Here's what some Thrivers had to say about their food sensitivities lifting after making progress!

1/30/2022
My stomach is slowly getting back to it's "normal" so can eat and drink a little bit more. My acne is finally pulling away as well!

2/15/2022
Last week most of the food sensitivities lifted, this week I had sleep improvement, and the fatigue is slowly lifting off as well. I can feel myself building back up.

3/14/2022
I'm out of my adjustment! Ate fried chicken and chips all weekend!!! Life's good! Hope everyone's doing well!

All About Sleep

It's common knowledge that sleep is very important when it comes to healing. However, sometimes we are not able to sleep. Maybe the body is buzzing, you feel wired, or there are a million different things going on in your mind that are keeping you up into the early morning hours. When you find yourself in a state of frustration, worry, and anxiousness from not being able to sleep, the next best thing you can do is similar to the way we approach all other symptoms of the hypersensitive nervous system. Stay cool, calm, and collected, because the less emotionally charged we are, the more our body is in a state of resting and digesting.

If you start getting frustrated, worried, or anxious, then the body will stay in sympathetic mode, and it will be nearly impossible to fall asleep. Growing up I found it extremely difficult to sleep, and I admit that my nighttime routine was less than optimal. All throughout high school I probably averaged five to six hours per night, even as I was playing multiple sports and keeping up with my grades. I would classify my old self as an extreme overthinker, especially during times when I suffered from concussions. I found that it was during the post-concussion phases (usually several weeks to several months after a concussion) that my sleep and overthinking were at their worst. I also used to stress myself out thinking that if I didn't get good sleep then the whole next day would be ruined, so without realizing it I put a lot of pressure on myself to "get to sleep." After getting sick, I tried my best to prioritize sleep and have "healthy sleeping habits." I had this seemingly perfect routine down where I would make sure my teeth were brushed, lights were off, and my eyes were closed by 9 pm. I had my blindfold on and earplugs in, however I was constantly stressed because in my mind this was the time to "perform" and get the restful sleep I longed for. The harder I tried to "fall asleep" the more awake I felt. When I tried my best to relax it would have the opposite effect and I felt more wired, simply because I was just trying way too hard.

Once I learned from my doctor in the hospital, I was no longer stressed about sleep, because I knew that stressing over it had zero benefits and only downsides. Over time, as I changed my relationship with sleep, it was easier and easier to get deep rest. My brain finally started shifting more into parasympathetic mode at nighttime as long as I caught myself before getting into a downward spiral of stress. I found I was getting eight to ten hours of sleep when I was making the most progress, but I wasn't very strict with my sleep. There is no exact amount of hours that I can tell you is right because we are all in different situations. I also found that during adjustment periods it was harder to sleep due to the flare-up of symptoms, and that's when I would practice the brain retraining exercise for chronic pain (coming up in the next section of this book). It's quite common to have the sleep schedule disrupted during the onset of an adjustment period as well as after the adjustment period (as the nervous system recalibrates itself). Overall, just like with any other issue, sleep will correct itself as you work on rebalancing the hypersensitive nervous system.

SLEEPING STRATEGIES AND TOOLS
*These are not necessary in order to recover, but they can help improve your quality of sleep. (I use all of these even to this day.)

Cool Showers
One strategy that helps many people get into a relaxed state is taking cool showers before bed. This forces your body to stimulate parasympathetic mode and "cool down" your nervous system. At first, you may feel your heart rate increase and feel stimulated, but shortly after the shower you will notice that you're more relaxed.

Blackout Curtains or Eye Mask
When you wear a sleeping mask or use blackout curtains, your body does not have to adjust to the changing light levels as much, which can make it easier for you to fall asleep. If you are exposed to light during the night, it can disrupt your sleep and make it harder for you to stay asleep. Having these tools blocks your eyes from all light.

Acupressure Mat
Acupressure mats are designed to apply pressure to these pressure points. This can help to relieve pain, improve circulation, and reduce stress and anxiety. All of these benefits can help you

to sleep better at night. In addition, the mat can also help to increase the production of endorphins, which are natural painkillers that can further improve your sleep quality.

Here's what some Thrivers had to say about their sleep improvements after making progress!

2/5/2022
Guys am not gonna lye im having some win pains ive got new muscles from carrying a shopping bag ...i must share by doing more yesterday this is the best sleep I've had in a year. Was a little wired getting to sleep but have the deepest rested sleep ever.

3/18/2022
First time in about 2 months since my fitbit said good sleep. Major win

1/29/2022
I got 8 hours of sleep for 3 nights in a row now and I feel euphoric

Dealing with Setbacks

On our path to recovery, we are going to have times of progress and times of setbacks (commonly known as dips). Will you have days where you feel down? Yes. Will you have days when you feel great? Absolutely. Recovery is a journey with ups and downs. These dips aren't setbacks, they are adjustment periods. As long as we don't overreact to adjustment periods and fall into that negative cycle that causes more symptoms - we won't experience these major setbacks. If we handle the adjustment period properly and use it as an opportunity to retrain the brain, we move in an upward trajectory. When we get discouraged and start doubting, then we veer off the course of recovery.

As you get better over time, you will have fewer and fewer symptoms. It's so crucial in the beginning to focus on not overreacting to the symptoms that you're feeling and keeping composure. Don't look at symptoms as something BAD, but as a scientific process that is occurring in your body. Use these periods of symptoms to rewire the way you perceive them.

For example, instead of responding with the following:

High heart rate → oh no, what health problem could this be…maybe I have x problem….can my heart handle all this stress….am I having a heart attack…?

React with:

High heart rate → This is just the nervous system being hypersensitive. I know it's going to calm down eventually. The more anxious I get about this the longer and more intense this experience will feel.

Overall, when you're focused on getting better, you'll find that your symptoms start to become less of a focal point in your life. You'll have more good days than bad days and eventually, the bad days will start to dissipate. That's what it means to be a Thriver, not a survivor. You're not letting chronic fatigue syndrome control your life - you're taking back control and living life on your terms.

Good Will

I'd like to create the opportunity to deliver this value to you during your reading or listening experience. In order to do so, would you be willing to help someone you don't know if it didn't cost you anything, but you never got credit for it? If so, I have a request to make on behalf of someone who is just like you or was like you a few years ago. You don't know them and likely never will. They are inexperienced and looking for information, but they don't know where to look. This is where you come in.

I can only help more people if they know about this information. Most people judge a book by its cover and its reviews. If you have found this book valuable so far, would you please take a brief moment right now and leave an honest review of the book? It will cost you zero dollars and less than 60 seconds. Your review will help one more Thriver learn about this information they otherwise would not have encountered and potentially change their life for the better. To make that happen, all you have to do is take less than 60 seconds to rate this book. If you're on audible hit the 3 dots on the top right of your device, click on rate and review, and then leave a few sentences about the book with the star rating. You can also go to the book page on Amazon or wherever you purchased this product and leave a review right on the page.

P.S. If you feel good about helping other Thrivers, I'm that much more excited to help you crush CFS in the coming chapters. You'll love the next strategy I'm about to go over.

Brain Retraining for Chronic Pain

If you suffer from chronic pain, look no further for a solution.

To give you an idea, my level of pain was above a 7/10 most of the time, and many times it was 10/10 (during these times I couldn't move because my entire body felt like it was on fire). I had headaches for years in addition to body aches and pains, burning sensations on my skin, and flu-like symptoms that flared up with increased activity.

Here is a simple exercise that has worked miracles for me and for many people around the world. It's also worth noting that I've created a video specifically breaking down what this exercise is and how it works on my YouTube channel, along with scientific data to back up everything I share about this exercise. The video is titled "Brain Retraining Can Cure Your Symptoms," and you can find it on my YouTube Channel "CFS Recovery." I'd highly recommend watching that video to fully understand what this exercise is all about and how to perform it.

In order for this exercise to work, it's important you understand the following:

- **You need to be dedicated and highly motivated when performing this exercise.**
- **You MUST perceive every episode of pain as an opportunity to rewire your brain and improve.**
- **You must perform this exercise consistently.**

I remember when I started really getting better, I would push myself to actually trigger symptoms so I could retrain them because now I was equipped with the proper tools to re-wire that pain. Prior to this knowledge, I would avoid pain at ALL costs, and when waves of pain did come it was a very neg-ative, demotivating experience because I felt paralyzed and help-less. Often times I would just lie down, close my eyes, put earplugs in, and wait for the pain to go away (which oftentimes took several hours). When I became good at this exercise it was kind of like having a "superpower" because I could lower the pain on command, and over time I would completely get rid of all the pain.

When I was in the hospital and my doctor first taught me about this exercise, I was still in a wheelchair. It was helping me immediately, but then maybe five or ten minutes later I would start feeling the headaches and body pain slowly start to come back. I would just keep doing the brain retraining exercise over and over again, and over time I had to do it less and less for it to have a lasting effect. You need to be relentless with this exercise at the beginning of your recovery because you really need to reawaken different neuropathways in your brain (the pathways that don't trigger chronic pain).

I'm not going to go into too much detail about this exer-cise because I've already broken this down in several YouTube videos that explain it a lot better along with visuals, but in a nut-shell, here are the FOUR basic steps for brain retraining when it comes to getting rid of chronic pain.

Step 1: Identify the Pain

Just close your eyes and take notice of where you're feeling the pain in your body. Is it in your head? Is it behind your eyes? You want to be very specific. For me, I used to get pain all over my body and especially in my legs and head. It felt like a burning sensation, so I imagined most of my body glowing red.

Step 2: Connect the Pain

Once you identify that pain, you want to connect that to your brain's pain centres. To do this, imagine there are glowing areas in your brain. Try to really feel how they're connected and associate that glow in your brain with the pain that you're feeling in your body.

Step 3: Slightly Expand the Pain Centres

Keeping your eyes closed, relax and start doing some slow, deep breathing and relax the body. Focus on expanding those pain centres in your brain ever so slightly. We want to gently expand the pain centres in the brain. At the same time, you're going to feel pain increase just a little bit, but keep in mind we don't want the glow to become too bright and the pain to get out of control.

Step 4: Dim the Pain Centres

We want to see the glow start to diminish. We want those epicentres to get smaller in your brain, and at the same time, because they're associated with the pain you're feeling in your body, the pain in your body will slowly start to dissipate.

At this point, you want to shift back and forth between step three and step four. The purpose of this exercise is not to completely remove the pain in the moment, but instead to teach your brain that it is in control, that it can actually affect the level of pain. Don't expect the pain to completely go away for the first several weeks, but do expect the pain to be less intense.

What we're looking for is for the intensity of pain to be lowered. Once you feel you're able to do that, you have now unlocked the power of brain retraining for chronic pain. The more you do this, the easier and faster you'll be able to lower the level of pain you're feeling. You may have to do this multiple times throughout the day. (I used to do this after parking my car, in the mall, in the washroom at a social gathering, really anywhere I could close my eyes for a couple of minutes and focus on this exercise.) Sometimes you only need two to three minutes to "reset" the pain levels to a more manageable level.

When to do this exercise: you need to do this when the pain is somewhat manageable. Do not wait until you're in a big flare-up.

How long should I do this for: do this at least 20 minutes per day, for AT LEAST 4 weeks before you say, "This doesn't work for me."

Keep in Mind

***If the pain gets worse afterward, that means you're doing something wrong. A common mistake is focusing *too much* on increasing the pain and glow of the "hot spots." The focus should be on lowering the level of pain and dimming the glowing red "hot spots."

I would highly recommend downloading the brain retraining guide for chronic pain, it's a PDF guide I've created that breaks all of this down into its simplest form and you can save it on your phone to reference when you do need to do this exercise. You can download it at www.cfsrecovery.co/pain.

BUILDING THRESHOLD

The third foundational step of recovery is building a threshold, and this is typically the longest step of recovery. This is where you're able to go out into the world, but you're still refining and fine-tuning things. People tend to feel fewer and fewer symptoms in this stage because they are much better, they're not home-bound or stuck in a bed all day. This is where having good habits comes in to play a massive role, but it can also be a grey area, because in the beginning, you can't quite live regularly like everybody else. We're trying to build that threshold for stress so your body will be able to handle more and more, and eventually, you'll be able to do everything else you used to do, if not more. There is no set end where you arrive at a destination and say "I'm done recovering." Now, this turns into a lifestyle where you're aware of treating your body better.

Here's what the transition from bedridden in the hospital to integrating back into society looked like for me. At first, my goal was just to move from my hospital bed into a wheelchair and get to the washroom on my own. I remember they even put a printed-out sign on the back of the wheelchair that said "Encourage Self-Propel." Transitioning from completely bedridden to moving around in a wheelchair was the most mentally challenging, worrying time of recovery because at that stage I knew the theory of what was happening with the body, but I had little evidence to support these theories other than putting faith in my doctor. As I recovered little by little, I gained more evidence that these strategies and tactics worked, so it was easier to have more confidence and continue doing the right things while avoiding many of the mistakes I made in the past. After about two weeks, I transitioned from moving around in a wheelchair to using a walker. I remember the first few days of doing any new activities were the most difficult due to my de-conditioned muscles.

When you are in certain positions for a long period of time, your muscles start to lose their ability to contract. Strength and endurance go down, and in my case my muscles shrunk to about one third of their original size. I had to keep this in mind whenever I would try to do more activity because not only was my nervous system hypersensitive, which triggered the burning and aching sensations all over, but my muscles were naturally getting sore. Walking fifty metres at that time was equivalent to me walking five thousand metres today. So, in addition to regular adjustment period symptoms my muscles legitimately felt as if I had done a workout, all from a simple walk across the room and back which was about a total of one hundred metres.

When I first got out of the hospital it felt like I had a new lease on life. For me, it would have been impossible to reach the "building threshold" stage until I experienced multiple mind shifts, learned exactly what's happening in my body, and learned how to properly deal with symptoms. Every time I had doubts when my symptoms would come back, I always had to bring my mind back to the principles of recovery.

Something else I found useful as I started to get better was this idea of a shifting scale. During recovery, doubt is very high while confidence is very low. I had tried so many different treatments and consulted with so many doctors in the past which only led to failure, I had low confidence and a high amount of doubt that these methods would work - luckily for me I had no choice but to believe in these methods my doctor showed me. If I were to draw a picture of two scales that represented both my confidence and doubt in recovery at the beginning, it would have looked like this:

Doubt in recovery methods   *Confidence in recovery methods*

However, as time went on and I saw more proof that these strategies worked, these scales started to shift in the opposite direction. Eventually, after dozens of progress cycles, getting through adjustment periods became a natural skill and it was easier and easier to keep up the momentum in recovery. Month over month I improved while putting less and less effort into "rewiring" my response to symptoms because it started happening automatically. About one year after being released from the hospital, the scale looked like this:

Doubt in recovery methods   *Confidence in recovery methods*

One of the examples I share in the <u>Recovery Jumpstart</u> program is the idea that picking up the skills needed to recover is kind of like surfing. I'd like to paint a picture for you.

Let's think of someone going out to surf properly for the first time. Imagine, they've tried doing it dozens of times in the past, but they just couldn't get the technique down. At some point after trying dozens if not hundreds of times, they get frustrated and decide it's time to go learn how to surf from a professional. Why do they want to surf?

It's been on their bucket list for years, it's been a dream of theirs, they've imagined how amazing it would be to glide on the water hundreds of times in the past, and the day has finally come for them to do their first surfing lesson with a master surfer.

Excitement sets in and the hopefulness is at an all-time high. The lesson begins, they learn the basic theory of waves, how the surfboard is built, how to balance, what to do, and what not to do. They spend some time preparing for the real surf, and they're told that most people wipe out a dozen times before their body finally grasps how to surf. So now after an hour, they're ready to swim out to the waves and, for the first time, they're going out there equipped with all the *theoretical knowledge* they need to surf.

They hop up on a board, catch their first wave, and wipe out. HARD. It takes a few minutes to swim back to the wave spot, they try again, but they fall over. This happens again, and again, and again. The frustration builds up because the knowledge they had just learned seems like it's not working. They know where they need to put their foot, how much to lean, but their body hasn't quite grasped it yet. The mind wants one thing, but the body does another.

What should they do? Should they just pack up, go home, and go back to trying to learn it on their own, or get back on the surfboard and continue trying?

That's right, they should try again.

It's just a matter of time until they get the hang of it.

It's just a matter of time before YOU get the hang of recovery.

The hardest part is the beginning of the journey, but once you get to a place where you understand how your nervous system has been overloaded with stimulus and the science behind your symptoms, building threshold is the part of recovery when you start integrating back into the world and rebuilding your life day by day, week by week, month by month.

I was lying down in my room all alone one night. I had just finished one of the busiest weeks of creating videos for clients. I thought to myself, I can't believe I was able to do this much activity without feeling symptoms. It felt amazing, liberating, and I finally felt like someone who could do activities at the level of a regular person. Just 12 months prior, I was lying in a hospital bed thinking that was my final chapter, so to be able to walk around, film, edit, and talk to clients multiple days in a row, it felt like I had a new life. The most important thing I did to be able to make that drastic change over a 12-month period *without any major relapses* was build my stress threshold.

How to create lasting change vs. temporary change

Stick to the Plan

When you're dealing with chronic fatigue syndrome, it can be really tempting to only do the things that make you feel better in the moment. You may be tempted to veer away from the plan when you're feeling good or to indulge in unhealthy habits when you're having a bad day. The truth is, if you want to create lasting change and beat chronic fatigue syndrome for good, you need to be consistent with the way you approach recovery, *both during the good days and bad days.*

No matter how you feel, no matter what's happening in your life, you need to control your response to the symptoms. A common mistake I see most people make is they don't stick with something long enough to see results. They'll get started, have a solid mindset, and remember to constantly retrain their response to symptoms. However, after a few weeks when they don't see massive changes, they get discouraged and stop it altogether. Then, they're back on the hunt looking for different solutions and the whole process repeats itself - this is what can drive people crazy.

It can be really tough to keep going when you don't feel like you're making any progress, but if you stick with the plan, eventually you will start to see results. If you're consistent with your approach, eventually you will see improvements in your symptoms and your quality of life. You won't see any massive changes day to day or week to week, which is why I tell people in the Recovery Jumpstart Program to only compare month to month. The improvements that happen will be so small that you will likely not realize they're happening until you take a step back and really think about what you were doing, how you were feeling, and most of all how you were responding to symptoms four weeks prior.

Patience

If you're used to being a go-getter who is always on the move, powering through any obstacles that come up in life, and putting your head down and willing your way through difficult situations, it can be really tough to slow down and be patient on this journey. Recovery is like nothing else in life, we can't force our way to the finish line, and in fact, there is no finish line. The marker of recovery is being able to do all the things you were previously able to do *before you got* sick, but you never arrive at some magical destination where you tell yourself, "I'm fully recovered." If you want to make lasting changes, you need to be patient with your approach. Sometimes we feel that resting is "wasted time" when in reality we are actually getting ahead by resting. Once you understand that taking rest days and (temporarily) skipping out on certain activities gives the body time to "recalibrate," you don't feel as bad on the slower days.

Another thing to keep in mind is the delayed effect of progress. You can be doing all the right things, working on the mindset, and following the path of recovery, however it's important to note that you won't see change overnight. Will you notice a big change once you have these mindshifts? Absolutely, but you may still feel a lot of the physical symptoms. Neuroplastic change takes time, but not as long as you might think. For example, people in the Recovery Jumpstart Program typically start feeling a massive shift in their perception of the illness, symptoms, and fatigue within the first two weeks. Does this mean they don't feel any symptoms at all? No, but because they are constantly being reminded that the symptoms are just triggered by an overactive nervous system and that there is no *real* danger, the symptoms are reduced. Once we get the ball rolling, typically 3-4 weeks in the program is when the results start compounding.

- If someone is having panic/anxiety attacks, they last a fraction of how long they used to last, and they are more or less physical sensations vs. feelings of impending doom.

- If someone has severe shortness of breath, now instead of just being able to walk to the kitchen and get food, they're able to walk outside to get some fresh air.

- If someone has a sensitivity to screens and headaches are triggered easily, they can now look at screens for forty-five minutes instead of five minutes.

This only happens shortly *AFTER* putting in the work needed. Whenever you feel you're doing all the right things and trying your best and progress seems to be at a standstill, ask yourself two questions:

- How am I responding to symptoms now?
- What was I doing and how was I responding to symptoms 30 days ago?

The answers to those questions will give you a clear indicator as to why you have or have not been making the progress you'd like to be making.

Living Life vs. Focusing All Attention on Recovery (you start thriving instead of surviving)

In the beginning stages of recovery, it absolutely has to be the priority of your life. However, once you learn the roadmap to recovery, gain traction, and make progress to the point where you can function again, it's important to remember that you also need to live your life. Being too focused on recovery can actually keep you stuck because you never allow yourself to have enjoyment and feel happiness. I encourage everyone in the program to pick up hobbies and exercise those creativity muscles because doing things outside of just recovery helps take your mind off tracking symptoms and constantly being on the lookout for things to retrain. One of the amazing things I found during recovery was videography. After living in my head for so long and just visualizing all the things I wanted to do, I had to get these overflowing ideas out and bring them to life. Eventually I started filming and editing one video per week, then two, then four. Then people started noticing, and I started getting paid to create videos. One thing led to another, and two years later I was busy running a video production company working with companies all around my city. Within three years of picking up a camera and filming, I started making YouTube videos about how to recover from chronic fatigue syndrome, and that channel took on a life of its own. (That's likely how you've found my work.) Now I'm able to reach people from all around the world and make a positive impact in their lives, and it all started with me picking up the camera shortly after getting out of the hospital.

The truth is we don't know where life will take us. If you're reading this right now, then you probably feel like you've been dealt a bad hand by life. However, I've always believed that it's not so much what happens to us in life, the most important thing is what we do with the cards we've been dealt. I didn't realize it when I was in the thick of my illness, but chronic fatigue syndrome was the springboard that catapulted me to new levels in life. I am now busier than I've ever been but I'm also the least stressed I've been, because I've learned to work efficiently rather than just trying to push through all the obstacles in life. I am able to balance work and play, intense focus and relaxation, and I no longer feel guilty for taking two or three days off of work to sit back and slow down. I feel like I get much more out of life now than before, not because of what I do but *how* I do things. Instead of surviving through the day, I thrive.

Thriving means living your life to the fullest, enjoying every moment, and creating lasting change. It's about more than just getting by day-to-day. It's about living with purpose and meaning, appreciating the "new lease on life" as I like to call it. That's how I felt walking out of the hospital on my own two feet just over four years ago. Prior to that moment, for about six months I never thought I would be independent again - I just didn't see how it was possible. I felt reborn, lucky, and so grateful just to be able to do simple things again. This is one of the most rewarding things I see in people who recover - I see that childlike curiosity come out in people, and they become so excited about the simplest of things because they've been deprived of them for so long. Simple things like going to dinner with friends, setting up a picnic on a nice day, or even just enjoying dinner with loved ones become that much more enjoyable (because they've likely pictured these scenes in their head thousands of times).

Creating lasting change is the key to thriving. It's not about making temporary changes that you'll quickly revert back to your old ways. Thriving is an important aspect of recovery that goes beyond just getting by day-to-day. To create lasting change and truly thrive, you need to make changes that will stick with you over time and work towards living a fulfilling and meaningful life.

Avoid These Mistakes

Overcomplicating Recovery

Overcomplicating recovery is one of the most common mistakes people make when trying to get a hypersensitive nervous system functioning properly again. When you're already feeling drained and exhausted, the last thing you need is to try and manage a million different things at once. Despite there being dozens of potential treatments out there, it's important to focus on one thing at a time and treat this as ONE problem - a hypersensitive nervous system issue. I know you've heard me say this over and over again throughout this book, but I cannot stress this enough. Start by simplifying the road to recovery and not falling into the trap of searching for a new solution every other week. Once you decide on what path you're going to take (hopefully the path I've set out in Recovery Jumpstart), stick to that path. Incorporating too many new things at once will only add to your stress levels and make your condition worse due to the stress of being overwhelmed.

I'm the perfect example of someone who made this crucial mistake in probably the worst way possible. I bounced from naturopath to naturopath and everything I was doing was to work on the symptoms, not the *actual root cause* of the symptoms. My naturopath did tell me we were doing this to heal my body as a whole, but he couldn't tell me exactly what was going on. At the end of the day, he was trying the next best thing he knew that might help me get better. You need to focus on getting your hypersensitive nervous system to a place where it functions normally again.

In the beginning, it can certainly be a journey of trial and error, but ultimately, it's worth it to continue crossing potential health issues off the list by doing tests and scans with doctors. If all your tests and scans come back as normal, then it is crucial you *believe* the facts the doctors are telling you. Sometimes we hope and pray the doctors tell us we have something because at least we'll be able to put a label on what we're feeling. When there's no official label, it leaves the door open for some kind of mystery illness that could potentially have no cure (at least that's what goes through our minds).

Trying to Do This on Your Own

I think in all of our lives, there are times when we can do things on our own, and there are times when we're better off hiring people who do this every day to help us, people who have walked down that path and experienced those hardships. Trying to do this all on your own can cost you years that you will never get back, so for situations like this, it would be wise to get extra help. You just can't leave recovery up to chance or luck. People who recover didn't just win the genetic lottery and one day something clicked inside their brain that allowed them to function normally again. No, they put in the work needed and followed the proven path to be successful on this journey.

At the end of the day, recovery is a formula, and it is replicable. If you just follow a few basic principles, recovery becomes inevitable. How would you like that? To know deep inside that eventually you are going to recover and it's only a matter of time for you to truly start living again. To know that even during the thick adjustment periods, when you're having headaches and flareups, you're going to be A-okay and you're going to come out of that adjustment period stronger than when you went in.

There are lots of really great people and programs out there that can help you. You don't have to work with me, but do get some guidance, and don't do this alone. When I say alone, I mean don't try doing this without someone who's been in your shoes before.

Here's an analogy to think about that will put all this into perspective.

Imagine you're traveling in a foreign city that you've never been to before. This isn't like any other city. Your family members, friends, and anyone you know personally hasn't visited or even heard of this place before. The streets are confusing, there are dead ends everywhere, and the buildings are so unrecognizable you might as well be on a different planet. You're in the middle of that city, and you need to catch a train that will take you back home. The only problem is you don't know where the train station is, and you don't have a clue which way to go. Would you rather:

A. Buy a GPS that tells you exactly where you need to go, allowing you to avoid all the detours and dead ends?

or

B. Continue to find your way through the city on your own?

Most people don't realize it, but they're stuck at a dead end trying to climb over it, and there's nothing on the other side. At the same time, they're afraid to "buy a GPS" because they've tried so many solutions in the past that didn't work, so the last thing they want to do is spend the last money they do have on yet another faulty GPS that only gets them two blocks further before becoming ineffective. I know I had serious trust issues after seeing over twenty-five doctors and specialists, naturopaths, and health professionals only to be told that I was "normal."

On rare occasions, someone would tell me they could fix me, and all I needed to do was buy more supplements or pay for more treatments. It cost me tens of thousands of dollars, some of which I didn't have and was putting on credit cards. Most people are in the same situation, desperate to find answers, however there are not many solutions out there. That's why I created the Recovery Jumpstart Program - it's a program filled with all the knowledge my doctor gave me that was the game changer in my recovery. I try to make it as simple and fail-proof as possible. If you join the program, show up to the calls, and follow the recovery roadmap (implement what you're learning), it's *extremely hard* to not make progress.

When you do make a decision to get that extra guidance, here's what you want to consider:

- You resonate with the program or person's story.
- You are actually ready for change.
- You are willing to commit to the program and follow through.

Again, you don't have to join my program, but do yourself a favour and just commit to *a* program where you have ongoing support and guidance from someone who's been on this journey before! Any time people want to get to the next level (whether in fitness, work, relationships, health, etc.), the easiest and fastest way to do that is by getting extra support.

That's why Michael Jordan, the greatest basketball player of all time, had a trainer.

That's why Tiger Woods, the greatest golfer of all time, had a trainer.

That's why Wayne Gretzky, the greatest hockey player of all time, had a trainer.

Without the extra help, you will prolong the process of recovery.

Expecting Symptoms to Go Away Too Soon

Thinking that your symptoms will go away quickly or believing that when they do start to go away they won't come back will lead to disappointment and cause lots of emotional stress due to disappointment. As you've learned earlier in this book, you will experience adjustment periods over and over again at different levels of recovery, so expect that. Perhaps you gain the ability to move around more, rebuild your social life, and gain traction in your recovery. There will come times when you introduce a new level of stimuli that triggers new symptoms - I experienced this dozens of times even when I started working full time again. Let's say you're able to get through a typical day symptom-free. This includes getting groceries, doing chores around the house, seeing friends, and even working part-time or full-time. If you were to start introducing exercise, it is likely that you would experience symptoms, however, getting to the next "level" requires the same approach mentioned previously. You handle the symptoms properly, allow your body time to adjust to this new level of stimuli, and soon you will be able to handle these new levels of exercise. If you're constantly living in fear of your symptoms coming back, then you're not really living at all, and you will likely bring about more symptoms. That's why in Recovery Jumpstart we teach people how to overcome symptoms, not just cope with them.

What Happens Next?

How the next 6 months go cannot be left up to chance, to nature, or to luck. At the end of the day, it's really up to you to determine your future.

The great thing is you don't need to change who you are inside. You'll still be the same person. You will just think in ways that lead to healthier and better outcomes for your life, plus you'll have knowledge about the human body that most people don't have. You'll know how to find balance much easier, and you'll learn to finally let go of things that are out of your control.

Chances are you've spent a lot of time and energy saying yes to so many opportunities in life and being a go-getter, even if it meant putting health to the side. Why not do something for yourself? Not for anybody else but YOU. No matter what's happened that has led you to where you are now, the solution is essentially the same. Give yourself the gift of health and commit to following what has been laid out in this book.

If you want extra help on your journey, I can help you. We accept members on an application basis. You can choose to apply, but there are limited spots available in the program because I can only work with so many people at once. If you do want to do this, fill out the application form, I'll look it over, we'll have an application call, and if you're the right fit for the program, then I would love to bring you into our community of Thrivers.

Just over 4 years ago, I was living a completely different life – one that was fuelled by fear, worry, and despair. Despite all the love and support around me, everything else seemed to be falling apart at the seams. And I'm not just saying that for dramatic effect – it legitimately was a living nightmare. I had no direction, no purpose other than to make it through the day, and no clue what the next few hours would bring. On the surface, everything looked great – I had a nice car, a good job, and a beautiful girlfriend – but on the inside, I was crumbling. And not just figuratively – I didn't even recognize who I was on the days that I *could* look in the mirror.

I'm so grateful that I didn't give up during those dark times and that I was able to find my way out of the darkness and into the light. I'm also grateful that everything happened the way it did because without going through all that, you wouldn't be reading this right now. More importantly, thousands of people wouldn't have seen all the helpful videos I post online about how to recover.

My Favourite Moment Throughout Recovery

When I was in Hawaii, standing on top of that mountain in Oahu, watching the sunrise, and feeling the wind on my face, I felt like I had just conquered the world. It was almost a metaphor for life, that no matter how bad of a situation you're in, no matter how horrible a place you've been and how deep in the trenches you are, if you continue to try your best and keep that vision of a brighter future alive, you'd be surprised where you can be 12 months from now. You can go from being bedridden to watching the sunrise from the top of a mountain (and be fully present in the moment without symptoms).

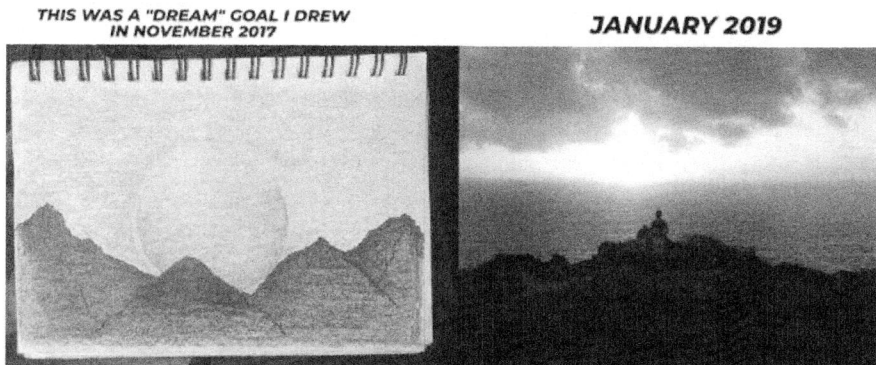

THIS WAS A "DREAM" GOAL I DREW IN NOVEMBER 2017   JANUARY 2019

When I was standing there, hundreds of memories flashed through my mind in a split second. All those letters I wrote to myself, all the drawings I made of watching the sunrise, all the visions I had of conquering this illness...to have that feeling of accomplishment and extreme gratitude for life - it made the journey worth it. And that's what I want other people to feel once they get their health back. That's what I want you to experience.

Repeat this manifesto daily to help instill within you the Thriver mentality.

I am a thriver

A survivor is a person who lived through hardship or disaster. A thriver is more than that. It is someone who not only goes through an exceptionally threatening life event, but shows subsequent growth because of the experience.

A thriver
-is a new kind of person
Patient . Composed . Dedicated . And Free.

A thriver
Believes in a future with thriving health
A future without chronic pain, suffering, and constraint

A thriver
-is in control of their destiny
They are able to persevere through challenges with unwavering commitment to better health

#thrivers
Define their own destiny
Prioritize recovery
Create their own progress
Impact the world

I am a thriver
And I Am Just One Mindshift away

Thank you for purchasing this book.

You chose this out of all the other books you could have read. Thanks for picking it! And thanks for reading it all the way through, I hope you found the recovery advice to be helpful.

To learn more about how to recover from CFS, visit my Youtube Channel called "CFS Recovery".

To get more hands on help on your recovery journey and work with people who are currently or have recovered, visit www.cfsrecovery.co/apply.

Printed in Great Britain
by Amazon

86063277R00047